Instructor's Manual
to accompany

The Professional Chef's
Techniques of Healthy Cooking
Second Edition

Instructor's Manual
to Accompany

The Professional Chef's
Techniques of Healthy Cooking
Second Edition

The Culinary Institute of America

Prepared by Lisa A. Lahey
with
Jennifer S. Armentrout

JOHN WILEY & SONS, INC.
New York, Chichester, Weinheim, Brisbane, Singapore, Toronto

Library of Congress Cataloging-in-Publication Data:

ISBN: 0-471-37955-7

Introduction

This instructor's manual has been prepared so that you can use it to suit a wide variety of curriculums and teaching styles. As you look through its pages, you will notice the following elements:

1.   Chapter Objectives

These have been provided to help you identify the learning objectives of each chapter and assist you in structuring your lessons.

2.   Lecture Outlines

We have compiled the contents of each chapter into major headings and subheadings, to act as a guide when preparing your classroom lectures. Use your own curriculum and class times to determine how much material you need for each day's lecture.

3.   Discussion Topics and Activities

There are a number of ways to help students delve deeper into any given topic. In this manual we have included a number of discussion topics and activities to generate in-class discussions, brainstorming sessions, written essay topics, and in- or out-of-class hands-on assignments.

4.   Keywords

You can use this feature to test mastery of the language used in the healthy kitchen during in-class question and answer sessions, or incorporate these terms into pop quizzes or a section in larger tests that you may administer to your class.

5.   Sample Study and Test Questions With Answers

These can be used either to review material or to test mastery. If you assign the short-answer questions as homework or include them on tests, you can look here for some elements that you might like to see in the responses that your students return to you.

6.   Glossaries

The nutrition and cooking glossaries are included here as a reference tool.

7.   Transparency Masters

In the back of the manual are several pages of helpful information and diagrams that can be photocopied onto transparencies for use on an overhead projector during your lectures.

Chapter One: The Language of Nutrition

Objectives

After reading and studying this chapter, the student will be able to:
1. Define the difference between nutrients and calories.
2. Name and identify the six basic nutrients: proteins, fats, carbohydrates, water, vitamins, and minerals.
3. Calculate the calories in foods from the four sources of calories: proteins, fats, carbohydrates, and alcohol.
4. Understand the USDA recommendations for daily calorie distribution.
5. Understand the roles that the basic nutrients play in maintaining good health.

Lecture Outline

Nutrients
Calories
      Empty calories/nutrient dense foods
Carbohydrates
      Simple carbohydrates
      Complex carbohydrates
Fiber
      Soluble fiber
      Insoluble fiber
Fat
      Saturated fat
      Monounsaturated fat
      Polyunsaturated fat
      Trans fat
      Omega-3 fatty acids
Cholesterol
      Low-density lipoprotein (LDL)
      High-density lipoprotein (HDL)
Protein
      Amino acids
      Complete/incomplete proteins
Water
Vitamins
      Water soluble
      Fat soluble
Minerals
      Macrominerals
      Microminerals

Activities/Assignments

1. List as many sources as you can think of for simple and complex carbohydrates; soluble and insoluble fiber; saturated fat, unsaturated fat, and trans fat; and complete and incomplete proteins.

2. Using a nutritional values handbook, practice calculating the calories in various foods from the four sources of calories.

3. Using recipes or prepared foods for which you have nutritional data, practice designing menus to meet USDA calorie distribution recommendations.

4. Read several food labels and determine which foods make the best choice for a healthy menu. Indicate if the product was nutritionally modified from its original form (reduced fat, low calorie, etc.).

Keywords

Amino acid-

Atherosclerosis-

Calorie (Kilocalorie, Kcal, or Calorie)-

Carbohydrate-

Cholesterol-

Complementary protein-

Complete protein-

Complex carbohydrates-

Dietary cholesterol-

Energy nutrients-

Enrichment-

Essential amino acid-

Essential nutrients-

Fat-

Fatty acid-

Fiber-

Fortification-

Glycogen-

High-Density Lipoprotein (HDL)-

Lipids-

Low-Density Lipoprotein (LDL)-

Macromineral (major mineral)-

Metabolism-

Micromineral (trace mineral)-

Mineral-

Monounsaturated fat-

Nutrients-

Polyunsaturated fat-

Protein-

Saturated fat-

Serum cholesterol-

Simple carbohydrates-

Trans fat-

Vitamin-

Water-

Sample Study and Test Questions

Discussion Topics and Essay Questions

1. Discuss the negative health effects of a diet high in saturated fats and cholesterol.

2. What steps can be taken to reduce the overall level of serum cholesterol in those who have been advised to reduce serum cholesterol?

3. Discuss the importance of both soluble and insoluble fiber in the diet, and also discuss ways to increase consumption of foods high in fiber.

True/False

T   Anemia is the result of an iron deficiency.

F   Fat soluble vitamins are excreted from the body each day.

F   Microminerals are less important to the proper functioning of the body than macrominerals.

T   Weight loss is achieved by altering the energy balance so that more energy is expended than consumed.

T   A person's level of activity will affect the number of calories needed to maintain his or her present weight.

F   No food provides all eight of the essential amino acids.

Short Answers

1. **What is an "empty calorie" food?**

    A food that provides energy, in the form of calories, without providing significant amounts of nutrients.

2. **Name 3 sources of soluble fiber.**

    Fruits, beans, vegetables, oats, and barley

3. **How many calories are in a gram of fat? A gram of carbohydrate? A gram of alcohol?**

    9;4;7

4. **What is glycogen?**

    The form in which animals and humans store glucose in the liver and muscles.

5. **Name some of the factors that affect cholesterol levels in the blood.**

    Age, weight, gender, genetics, activity level, stress, and consumption of foods high in saturated fats, trans fats, and cholesterol.

Additional Resources

Drummond, Karen Eich. *Nutrition for the Foodservice Professional*. 3rd edition. New York: Van Nostrand Reinhold, 1997.

Hodges, Carol A. *Culinary Nutrition for Food Professionals*. 2nd edition. New York: Van Nostrand Reinhold, 1994.

Chapter Two: The Pyramids

Objectives

After reading and studying this chapter, the student will be able to:
1. Identify average American diet-related health problems.
2. Define the dietary guidelines for the USDA Food Guide Pyramid, the Mediterranean Pyramid, and the Vegetarian Pyramid.
3. Understand the differences and similarities between the three food guide pyramids.
4. Name and identify the 1995 USDA Dietary Guidelines for Americans.

Lecture Outline

The average American diet
    Nutritional imbalance
    Life Style
    Disease
USDA pyramid
    Purpose
    Grain-based foods
        Servings per day
        Caloric intake per day
        Food included in the group
    Fruits and vegetables
        Servings per day
        Caloric intake per day
        Food included in the group
    Dairy
        Servings per day
        Caloric intake per day
        Food included in the group
    Proteins
        Servings per day
        Caloric intake per day
        Food included in the group
    Fats and oils
        Servings per day
        Caloric intake per day
        Food included in the group
Mediterranean pyramid
    Origins
    Dietary guidelines
Vegetarian pyramid
    Origins
    Dietary guidelines

Activities/Assignments

1. Design daily meal plans based on each pyramid.

Keywords

Atherosclerosis-

Diabetes-

Mediterranean food pyramid-

USDA food pyramid-

Vegetarian food pyramid-

Sample Study and Test Questions

Discussion Topics and Essay Questions

1. Discuss the health problems to which the average American diet contributes.

2. Discuss the differences between the three food guide pyramids.

True/False

T   According to USDA recommendations, 55 to 60 percent of daily calories should come from carbohydrates.

F   The average American diet is high in fiber.

T   According to the USDA, fruits and vegetables should make up the second largest component of your diet.

T   The Mediterranean Pyramid suggests that red meat should only be consumed a few times per month.

F   Olive oil is a saturated fat.

Short Answer

1. **Explain the difference between the USDA Food Guide Pyramid, the Mediterranean Pyramid, and the Vegetarian Pyramid.**

   The USDA Food Guide Pyramid emphasizes daily servings and portion sizes for different types of foods, while the Mediterranean Pyramid prioritizes food choices in order to maximize the benefits of certain foods. The ADA Vegetarian Pyramid substitutes alternate protein sources for the traditional meats, fish, and poultry found in the USDA Pyramid. Other than this difference, the Vegetarian Pyramid is structured the same as the USDA Food Guide Pyramid.

2. **Identify the 1995 USDA Dietary Guidelines for Americans.**

   1. Eat a variety of foods every day.

   2. Balance the food you eat with physical activity—maintain or improve your weight.

   3. Choose a diet with plenty of grain products, vegetables and fruits.

   4. Choose a diet low in fat, saturated fat and cholesterol.

   5. Choose a diet moderate in sugars.

   6. Choose a diet moderate in sodium.

   7. If you drink alcoholic beverages, do so in moderation.

3. **List 6 major American health problems that are diet-related.**

   Obesity, cancers, Type2 diabetes, atherosclerosis, stroke, and heart disease

4. **How often does the USDA revise its dietary guidelines?**

   Every 5 years

5. According to the USDA what percentage of daily calories should come from carbohydrates, fat, and protein?

Carbohydrates: 55 to 60 percent

Fat: 30 percent

Protein: 12 to 15 percent

Chapter Three: The Elements of Flavor

Objectives

After reading and studying this chapter, the student will be able to:
1. Understand the significance of all the senses in relation to flavor.
2. Understand what variables affect perception of flavor.
3. Explain the importance of layering flavors in healthy cooking.

Lecture Outline

Seeing flavor
      Color
      Plate presentation
Hearing flavor
      Texture
Smelling flavor
      Importance of smell to the sense of taste
Feeling flavor
      Mouth feel
      Texture
Tasting flavor
      Taste receptors
      Importance of temperature
Flavor perception
      Variables
            Environment
            Mood
            Health
      Describing flavor
            The words we choose
      Flavor ranges
Building flavor
      Ingredient attributes
      Balancing flavor
      Contrasting flavor
      Importance of cooking time
      Importance of ingredient sequence

Activities/Assignments

1. Conduct a taste test with a variety of aromatic ingredients (fresh herbs, berries, citrus, wine). Have participants taste first with their noses pinched shut, then again normally to explore the effect of aroma on flavor perception.

2. Select several dishes and deconstruct them to explore how flavor is developed in each one.

3. Discuss a personal "flavor memory."

4. Select a particular food and describe its flavor profile.

Keywords

Balance-

Complement-

Contrast-

Finish-

Flavor ranges-

Flavor layering-

Flavor profile-

Umami-

Sample Study and Test Questions

Discussion Topics and Essay Questions

1. Discuss how each of the five senses are important in flavor perception.

2. How are flavor ranges useful in understanding flavor relationships?

True/False

F   When creating a dish, balance is always important.

F   Taste is the most important component of flavor.

F   Of the two senses, taste and smell, taste will help you the most in distinguishing between a lemon and a lime.

T   All five senses contribute to our perception of flavor.

T   Humans are physically able to detect hundreds of different aromas.

F   Hot and cold foods should never be served on the same plate.

Short Answer

1. **What variables affect flavor perception?**

    Combination of ingredients, timing of preparation, the order in which ingredients are added to a dish during cooking, the temperature at which the food is served, mood, health, and environment

2. **What is the optimal service temperature range for flavor perception and why?**

    Flavor perception is heightened when foods are served between 72°C and 105°C because we are most sensitive to taste at these temperatures.

3. **What are the five senses that contribute to flavor perception?**

    Sight, sound, smell, touch, and taste

4. **Why is flavor perception subjective?**

    People vary in their ability to sense and interpret flavor cues.

5. **Why are ingredients added at different times during the cooking process?**

    To maximize flavor and ensure that each ingredient is cooked just enough.

Chapter Four: Fruits and Vegetables, Grains and Legumes

Objectives

After reading and studying this chapter, the student should be able to:
1. Explain why plant foods are the foundation of a healthy diet.
2. Understand what factors lead to nutrient loss in plant foods.
3. Describe the proper storage conditions for fruits, vegetables, grains and legumes.
4. Explain the different classifications of vegetarians and their specific dietary concerns.

Lecture Outline

Fruits and vegetables
    Nutritional value
    Purchasing
        Quality
        Quantity
    Storage
        Compatibility of different fruits and vegetables
        Temperature and humidity
        Length of storage
    Preparation
        Timing
        Cooking techniques
Fruit and vegetable integration
    Choosing the fruits and vegetables most appropriate for a particular dish
    Flavors that connect fruits and vegetables to other components in the dish
    Fruit and vegetable juices
Grains
    Purchasing
        Processed grains
        Milling processes
    Storage
        Length of storage
        Rancidity
    Preparation
        Culinary applications
        Varieties
        Cooking techniques
Ancient grains
Legumes
    Purchasing
    Storage
        Length of storage

Preparation
        Culinary applications
        Varieties
        Cooking techniques
Nuts and seeds
        Nutritional significance
        Purchasing
        Storage
        Culinary applications
Phytochemicals
        Benefits
        Sources
Plant-based menu items
        Consumer popularity
        Importance to menu
How to approach development of these items on the menu
        Appearance
        Flavor
Vegetarians
        Three types
        Hidden meat products

Activities/Assignments

1.	Design three to five entrées with integrated vegetable and starch components.

2.	Design a multi-course vegetarian meal.

Keywords

Alternivore-

Antioxidants-

Batch cooking-

Carotenoids-

Ethylene gas-

Free radicals-

Lacto-ovo vegetarian –

Lacto vegetarian-

Lycopene-

Oligosaccharides-

Phytochemicals-

Vegan vegetarian-

Vegetable integration-

Sample Study and Test Questions

Discussion Topics and Essay Questions

1. Explain the cooking procedures that will result in the greatest nutrient retention for vegetables.

2. Explain vegetable integration and discuss some ways in which to implement the technique.

3. Discuss why it is important to become familiar with different types of grains and grain products.

True/False

T   Bananas accelerate the ripening and spoilage of some fruits.

F   Some vegetables contain cholesterol.

F   Couscous is a whole grain.

T   Soaking beans prior to preparation results in the leaching of nutrients.

F   Highly refined flours will spoil faster than whole grain flours.

Short Answer

1. **What factors cause nutrient loss in vegetables?**

   Exposure to light, moisture, heat, metals, alkalis, and acidic conditions as well as age will cause nutrient loss.

2. **Give four examples of fruits that produce ethylene gas.**

   Apples, bananas, avocados, and melons

3. **Why is important to keep ethylene producing fruits away from certain fruits?**

   Some fruits are ethylene sensitive. The gas will cause them to ripen and spoil at a much faster rate.

4. **Why is blanching a beneficial step in vegetable preparation?**

   Blanching will stop enzymatic reactions that cause nutrient loss.

5. **Name some healthy cooking techniques that can be applied to vegetables.**

   Grilling, stir-frying, broiling, roasting, steaming, pan steaming, and microwaving

6. **What health benefits are phytochemicals linked to?**

   They reduce the risk of heart disease and cancer.

7. **Why is it important to remove the leafy tops from vegetables such as beets before storage?**

   After harvest, leaves continue to absorb nutrients from the root.

Chapter Five: Cooking with Less Fat

Objectives

After reading and studying this chapter, the student will be able to:
1. Discuss the difference between saturated, monounsaturated, polyunsaturated, and hydrogenated fats.
2. Understand the pros and cons of different fat substitutes on the market today.
3. Understand the function of fat in baking and cooking.
4. Understand how to cook with less fat, but maintain flavor.

Lecture Outline

Functions of fat
      Cooking
      Baking
Caloric content of fat
Types of fat
      Saturated
            Characteristics
            Sources
            Health benefits
      Monounsaturated
            Characteristics
            Sources
            Health benefits
      Polyunsaturated
            Characteristics
            Sources
            Health benefits
      Hydrogenation
            Trans fats
Cooking oils
      Varieties
      Storage
      Purchasing
Reducing fat in cooking
      Identify its function
      Low fat ingredients
            Poultry
            Meat
            Fish
      Cooking methods
      Flavored oils
            Ground spice oils
            Fresh root oils

Activities/Assignments

1. Conduct a comparative tasting of various olive oils.

2. Choose a high- to moderate-fat recipe and experiment in the kitchen with various ways to reduce the fat.

Keywords

Extra-virgin olive oil-

Hydrogenated fats-

Infused oil-

Monounsaturated fat-

Olestra-

Olive-pomace oil-

Omega-3 fatty acids-

Polyunsaturated fats-

Protein-based fat substitute-

Saturated fats-

Trans fats-

Virgin olive oil-

Sample Study and Test Questions

Discussion Topics and Essay Questions

1. Discuss the controversy surrounding Olestra.

2. Describe the process in creating a low-fat recipe.

3. What functions does fat fulfill in baking and what are some likely substitutes?

4. Discuss the functions of fat in cooking.

True/False

F   Saturated fats have a higher smoking point than polyunsaturated and

monounsaturated fats.

T   Walnuts are a good source of omega-3 fatty acids.

F   Light olive oil has less fat than other olive oils.

T   Squid is high in cholesterol.

F   Poultry skin should always be removed before cooking.

Short Answer

1. **What are some of the important functions fat fulfills in cooking and baking?**

   Mouth feel, blending of flavors, improved appearance, tenderizes, leavens, retains moisture, texture, transfers heat, emulsifies and thickens, yields a crisp texture

2. **What are some typical sources of saturated fats?**

   Butter, lard, and tropical oils

3. **How can you tell which hydrogenated fats have less trans fats?**

   The softer the fat is at room temperature the less trans fats it contains.

4. **What are the four grades of olive oil and what do they indicate?**

   "Extra-virgin" is the most pure. It is the finest and most expensive and is generally used in cold preparations. "Virgin" is the next best grade and is produced in much the same way as extra-virgin. "Olive oil" is generally used for cooking because it lacks the delicate flavors of the first two grades. The lowest grade is "olive-pomace" and it is extracted from the pulp after extra-virgin and virgin grades have been extracted.

5. **What is the difference between Asian and Middle Eastern sesame oils?**

   Asian sesame oil is extracted from toasted seeds and has a great deal of flavor. Middle Eastern sesame oil is light in color and is used primarily because it has a high smoking point.

6. **Why is it a good practice to cook stocks, soups, stews and braises a day in advance?**

   Flavor will continue to develop and fat removal is easy as the fat rises to the surface and solidifies.

7. **When replacing reduced-fat milk products for whole milk, why does curdling commonly occur and how can this be avoided?**

Reduced fat milk does not have enough fat to prevent the proteins from binding together (coagulating). This may be avoided by using gentle heat and adding the milk at the last minute.

8. **Why can it be hazardous to infuse oils with garlic and herbs?**

Oil creates an anaerobic environment that facilitates the growth of certain pathogens.

9. **What types and cuts of meat, fish and poultry are lower in fat?**

In general, loin and round cuts from meats and poultry breasts are the leanest choices. Choosing meats according to USDA standards is a reliable way to judge lean meat. Another way to select leaner meats is to buy according to breed; Limousin, Belgian Blue, Chianina and Chiangus breeds can be substantially lower in fat and calories than standard USDA Choice. Fish is an excellent choice low in saturated fats and calories and high in omega-3 fatty acids. Most shellfish contains the same advantages as fish, although some shellfish, such as squid, are very high in cholesterol.

Chapter Six: Moderating Salt

Objectives

After reading and studying this chapter, the student will be able to:
1.   Explain the health risks associated with a high sodium diet.
2.   Know where to look for hidden sources of sodium.
3.   Understand how to reduce reliance on sodium in cooking.
4.   Understand how to use different salt substitutes.

Lecture Outline

Health effects
>   Hypertension

Hidden sources of sodium
>   Processed Foods

Reducing salt in cooking
>   How to add salt during cooking
>   Serving temperatures
>   Benefits of using high sodium ingredients

Types of salt

Natural flavors
>   Building flavor
>   Combining and contrasting flavors
>   Herbs and spices
>   Aromatic ingredients
>   Chiles
>   Pungent ingredients
>   Acidic foods

MSG
>   Controversy
>   As a salt substitute

Activities/Assignments

1.   Visit a local supermarket and peruse the nutrition labels on various products for

sodium content. Try to identify products you believe will be low in sodium, then

check the label. Discuss your findings.

Keywords

Canning and pickling salts-

Iodized salt-

Kosher salt-

MSG-

Potassium chloride-

Rock salt-

Sea salt-

Table salt-

Sample Study and Test Questions

Discussion Topics and Essay Questions

1. Discuss the link between sodium and hypertension.

2. Explain the purpose of salt in relation to flavor and discuss possible alternatives.

3. Discuss and explain the controversy surrounding MSG.

True/False

T   Salt is more effective as a flavoring when added incrementally throughout the cooking process rather than all at once.

F   Salt is less prominent to the taste buds when served at cooler temperatures.

T   Prepared horseradish and mustard may contain added salt.

F   Most Americans do not have enough salt in their diets.

T   MSG contains 1/3 the amount of sodium in salt.

F   Kosher salt may be substituted equally for table salt.

Short Answer

1. **In what type of individuals is salt likely to affect health?**

    People who have a preexisting hypertensive condition

2. **What is the FDA-recommended daily intake for sodium?**

    Under 2400 mg/day which is just over 1 teaspoon

3. **Why do many chefs prefer kosher salt over table salt for cooking?**

    Kosher salt dissolves more readily and adheres better to food.

4. **Name five ingredient alternatives to salt.**

    Herbs and spices, aromatic ingredients, chiles, pungent ingredients, and acidic

    ingredients

5. **What is MSG?**

    Monosodium glutamate, which is the sodium salt of glutamic acid, a common

    amino acid. It naturally occurs in almost all foods.

Chapter Seven: Sweeteners

Objectives

After reading and studying this chapter, the student will be able to:
1. Define different types of sugars and sweeteners.
2. Understand the function sugars fulfill in cooking and baking.
3. Discuss ways of replacing sugar in recipes.
4. Understand the controversy surrounding non-caloric sweeteners.

Lecture Outline

Refined sugar
      Health
Natural sugars
      Fruits
      Benefits
      Flavor
      Sweet spices
      Caramelization
Function of sugar in a recipe
      Color
      Viscosity
      Inhibits staling
      Facilitates fermentation process
Forms of sugar
      Crystal
      Liquid (invert)
Flavors and uses of different sugars
      Molasses
      Honeys
      Maple sugar and syrup
      Invert sugars
      Granulated sugar
      Brown sugar
      Raw sugar
      Palm sugar
Hidden sugars
      Processed and refined foods
Non-caloric sweeteners
      Types
      Uses in the kitchen
      Health

Assignments/Activities

1. Conduct a tasting of various types of honeys and other sweeteners.

2. Cut two pieces from a single fruit (apple, banana, peach, pineapple). Sauté or roast one piece until it caramelizes. Compare the flavors of the raw and caramelized pieces.

3. Allow a spoonful of a sweetened dessert, such as ice cream or sorbet, to melt on your tongue. Notice whether or not the dessert seems to become sweeter as it melts.

Keywords

Acesulfame-potassium-

Aspartame-

Caramelization-

Empty calories-

GRAS-

Palm sugar-

Refined sugar-

Saccharin-

Sucralose-

Turbinado sugar-

Sample Study and Test Questions

Discussion Topics and Essay Questions

1. Discuss the reasons why it is beneficial to reduce the amount of sugar in your diet.

2. Define the different types of sugars and what type of applications each is best suited for.

3. Discuss the controversy and health risks people feel are associated with non-caloric sweeteners.

True/False

T   Honey is a refined sugar.

F   Sugar causes diabetes.

F   Liquid and crystal sugars are basically the same and are interchangeable.

T   Invert sugars inhibit crystallization.

F   Brown sugar and raw sugar are the same thing.

T   People are more sensitive to sweet tastes at warm temperatures.

Short Answers

1. **How are refined sugars made?**

    Simple carbohydrates found in other foods are concentrated and purified to make

    refined sugar.

2. **What is caramelization?**

    When heat is applied to sugar, a chemical reaction causes the sugar to darken and

    take on complex flavors.

3. **How are honeys usually named?**

    They are usually named for the predominant flower the pollen came from.

4. **Why are products that are made with liquid sugars moister and chewier than**
    those made with crystal sugar?

    Liquid sugars attract water molecules.

5. **What ingredient is added to confectioners' sugar and why?**

    Cornstarch is added to prevent the sugar from clumping.

6. **Why are non-caloric sweeteners non-caloric?**

    These types of sweeteners are extremely concentrated. Such a small amount

    needs to be added to a product to make it sweet that it yields no calories.

Chapter Eight: Beverages

Objectives

After reading and studying this chapter, the student will be able to:
1. Name and discuss the health benefits associated with alcohol.
2. List the health drawbacks associated with alcohol.
3. Understand the importance of nonalcoholic beverages on the menu.

Lecture Outline

Alcohol
    Health
        Alcoholism
        Social problems
        Benefits
            Heart disease
            Moderation
            Recommended daily amounts
            Red wine
                Antioxidants
    Cooking with alcohol
        Applications
        Evaporation
Beverage promotion
    Nonalcoholic beverages
    Alcoholic beverages

Activities/Assignments

1. Design a beverage menu that emphasizes nonalcoholic drinks as much as alcoholic drinks.

2. Develop 5 ideas for unusual, appealing, nonalcoholic cocktails.

Keywords

Antioxidants-

Cirrhosis-

Evaporation-

French paradox-

HDL-

LDL-

Phenolic compounds-

Tannins-

Sample Study and Test Questions

Discussion Topics and Essay Questions

1. Discuss why it is important to have a beverage menu with nonalcoholic selections.

2. Discuss ways in which you might promote you beverage menu.

3. Explain the health benefits associated with drinking alcohol.

True/False

F Countries with the lowest rates of wine consumption also have the lowest rates of heart disease.

F The amount of calories added to a dish through alcohol is solely dependant on the amount of alcohol added.

T Body cells are composed mostly of water.

F Prolonged cooking will evaporate all alcohol that is present in a dish.

F Red wine is the only alcoholic beverage that can help prevent heart disease.

Short Answer

1. **What is considered a moderate amount of alcohol to consume so that the benefits are gained with none of the drawbacks?**

   Less than 2 drinks per day; one drink equals 12 fluid ounces of beer, 5 fluid ounces of wine, or 1½ fluid ounces of liquor

2. **Why is red wine the most beneficial alcoholic beverage?**

   Red wine contains phenolic compounds, which are antioxidants. They help to lower the level of LDL and increase levels of HDL. They also aid in the prevention of blood clots and suppress tumors.

3. **What factors affect the rate of alcohol evaporation in cooking?**

   Temperature, length of exposure to heat, and the surface area of the pot

4. **What is the French Paradox?**

   The term used to describe the contradiction between the low heart disease rate in France and the high consumption of fat.

Chapter Nine: The Techniques of Healthy Cooking

Objectives

After reading and studying this chapter, the student should be able to:
1. Understand which cooking techniques promote a healthy diet.
2. Explain ways to prevent nutrient loss in foods.
3. Describe how to maximize flavor in different healthy cooking techniques.

Lecture Outline

Cooking guidelines
 Nutrient retention
  Variables
Sautéing
 Benefits
 Dry sautéing
 Preparation of foods prior to cooking
 Seasoning and flavor
 Sauces
 Deglazing
 Equipment
  Shape of the pan
  Material of construction
   Different metals
   Nonstick coating
Stir-frying
 Benefits
 Procedure
  Preparation of ingredients
  Amount of cooking oil
 Equipment
Grilling
 Benefits
 Applications
  Types of foods and menu items
 Procedure
  Marination
  Precooking
  Flavors
  Wood chips
  Dry herbs
  Herb stems
 Sauces

Broiling
- Benefits
- Applications
  - Gratin

Roasting/baking
- Benefits
- Applications
- Carryover cooking time
- Crust coatings

Smoke roasting
- Benefits
- Procedure
- Aromatics
- Marination

Steaming
- Benefits
- Applications
- Procedure
- How to incorporate flavor
- En papillote
  - Procedure
  - Applications
- Sauces

Shallow poaching
- Benefits
- Procedure
- Applications
- Sauces

Deep poaching/simmering/boiling
- Benefits
- Procedure
- Applications
- Temperatures

Stewing/braising
- Benefits
- Applications
- Procedure
- Sauce
- Techniques
  - Fully submerged
  - Partially covered

Microwave cooking
- Reheating application
- Benefits
- Procedure

Keywords

À la minute-

Carcinogen-

Carryover cooking-

Deglazing-

Dry sautéing –

En papillote-

Fond-

Gratin-

Presentation side-

Sample Study and Test Questions

Discussion Topics and Essay Questions

1. Discuss why flavor is a challenge in healthy cooking.

2. Explain what make a cooking technique healthy.

3. List ways to retain nutrients in cooking and explain ways in which nutrients are lost.

True/False

F   Boiling foods causes nutrients to be retained.

F   If you sauté or stir-fry properly, the amount of oil added to the pan will not decrease the healthy aspects of these cooking techniques.

T   When sautéing, foods should be left alone to brown properly so they will not stick to the pan.

T   Marinating foods prior to grilling may reduce the presence of carcinogens.

T   Fat should be poured off a roasting pan before deglazing.

F   It is necessary to oil the paper when cooking en papillote.

F   Deep poaching is done between 185°F and 200°F.

Short Answer

1.   **What variables may cause a loss of nutrients in foods?**

Nutrients are lost when foods are exposed to light, air, or excessively high heat and when they are overcooked, cooked in too much liquid, or in alkaline or very acidic conditions.

2.   **What is one of the best ways to minimize nutrient loss?**

Prepare foods as close to cooking time as possible.

3.   **Why are stewing and braising considered to be nutrient-conservative cooking methods?**

The cooking liquid in these techniques, which captures lost nutrients, is used as the sauce.

4.   **What types of foods should be precooked prior to sautéing?**

Denser ingredients such as carrots

5.   **What does it mean to season a pan?**

A pan, typically cast iron, is heated with a film of oil. The oil penetrates the surface of the pan and seals the pores in the metal, creating a nonstick coating.

6.   **What is the major difference between broiling and grilling?**

In grilling the heat source is below the product while in broiling the heat source is above.

7.   **Why is carryover cooking an important concept to remember when roasting?**

It is important to remember a certain amount of cooking occurs after the product has been removed from the oven because it will prevent overcooking.

8.   **What function does a crust coating provide in baked items?**

It will help to prevent them from drying out.

9. **Why is the shape of a sauté pan important?**

The flat bottom provides a cooking surface, while the sloping sides encourage any

juices released into the pan to reduce rapidly, forming the fond.

Chapter Ten:
Agricultural Issues in Ingredient Selection

Objectives

After reading and studying this chapter, the student will be able to:
1.   Understand the meaning of sustainable agriculture.
2.   Understand what "organically grown" means.
3.   Discuss the pros and cons of biotechnology.
4.   Define irradiation and understand its effects.

Lecture Outline

Sustainable agriculture
       The philosophy behind it
       Problems it addresses
       Maintaining balance
Organic farming
       USDA guidelines
            Produce
            Livestock
Labeling on organic processed foods
       Benefits
            Health
            Consumer popularity
Free-range poultry
       USDA requirements
       Benefits
            Flavor
            Health
            Consumer popularity
Plant biotechnology
       Pros
       Cons
       Product examples
       Labeling
Heirloom seeds and plants
       Conservation
       Flavor
Irradiation
       Uses
       Benefits
       Nutrient loss
       Labeling

Activities/Assignments

1. Conduct interviews with people to determine public attitudes in your area regarding organic foods, irradiation, and/or biotechnology.

2. Visit the produce sections of local supermarkets to see how much produce is labeled as either organic or irradiated. Talk to the produce manager about demand for these products.

3. Visit local butchers to determine demand for organic and free-range meats and poultry. Survey other foodservice operators who offer organic and free-range foods to see how well they sell.

4. Visit an organic farm. Get to know your local farms and purveyors.

Keywords

Bioengineering-

Biotechnology-

Cross-breeding-

Free-range-

Heirloom plants-

Integrated pest management-

Irradiation-

Organic-

Radura-

Sustainable agriculture-

Sample Study and Test Questions

Discussion Topics and Essay Questions

1.   Explain what irradiation means and the controversy surrounding it.

2.   Discuss the controversy surrounding biotechnology.

3.   Explain the purpose of sustainable agriculture.

4.   What are heirloom seeds and why are they significant?

True/False

F   Adverse farming methods generally only affect a small area.

F   Organic livestock must be provided sunlight and access to the outdoors.

T   For a product to be labeled organic, 95% of its ingredients must be certified organic.

T   All living things are similar at the level of DNA.

F   Irradiation makes food radioactive.

Short Answer

1. **Give a brief definition of sustainable agriculture.**

    Sustainable agriculture uses agricultural practices that benefit the health of the environment and the health of society.

2. **What are some of the problems that have been caused by agricultural practices in the last decade?**

    Topsoil depletion, excessive water and energy consumption, decrease in air quality, contamination of the ground water.

3. **What is IPM and how does it work?**

    IPM stands for Integrated Pest Management. It is a variety of farming strategies used to decrease the use of chemical pesticides. These strategies include using predatory insects for pest control, growing pest-resistant crops, and monitoring environmental conditions to predict pest outbreaks.

4. **What are the guidelines for free-range poultry?**

    They must have access to the outdoors.

5. **What are some of the positive applications of biotechnology?**

    Biotechnology can create plants that are resistant to frost, disease, drought, pests, and herbicides. It can improve nutrition, productivity, and shelf life.

6. **What foods are approved for irradiation?**

    Dried seasonings, fruits, grains, vegetables, poultry, beef, and lamb are approved for irradiation.

Chapter Eleven: Menu and Recipe Development

Objectives

After reading and studying this chapter, the student sill be able to:
1.   Discuss techniques for surveying the market.
2.   Understand how to set standards for menu and recipe development.
3.   Understand how to develop a healthy menu.

Lecture Outline

Examining the market
       Customer preference
              Market survey
              Using the knowledge of your staff
              Sales reports
              Developing a questionnaire
Standards for menu development
       Customer traits
              Age
              Gender
              Lifestyle
Menu planning parameters
       Nutrient ranges
              FDA daily values
                     Calories per day per meal
       Fat
       Sodium
       Cholesterol
Breakfast
       Calorie ranges
       Healthy choices
              Food
              Beverages
Brunch
       Calorie ranges
       Breakfast and lunch selections
Lunch
       Calorie ranges
       Portion sizes
       Menu selections
Dinner
       Calorie ranges
       Multiple courses
Portion size
       Reduce portion sizes of meat, fish and poultry

Increase portion size of vegetables, fruits, grains and legumes
Customer perception
Standardizing recipes
Recipe development
    Existing recipes
        Nutritional evaluation
    Making recipe alterations
        Cooking technique
        Substitution of ingredients
        Garnishes
        Portion size
    Original recipes

Activities/Assignments

1. Design a sample questionnaire for a market survey.

2. Design menus that fall within pre-set parameters such as those within this chapter.

3. Modify a recipe on paper, then test your approach in the kitchen.

Keywords

Daily values-

Nutrient ranges-

Portion sizes-

Standard recipe-

Sample Study and Test Questions

Discussion Topics and Essay Questions

1. What is the first step in creating a healthy menu and how would you approach gaining this information?

2. Discuss the different ways to develop recipes.

3. Explain the things you would look at when nutritionally evaluating a recipe.

4. Discuss the importance of standard recipes.

True/False

T   It is good practice to reduce the portion size of high-fat foods.

T   When substituting ingredients in a recipe, function and flavor are the most important considerations.

T   Cocoa powder can be used as a substitute for chocolate.

T   High-calorie and high-fat foods do not have to be completely eliminated in healthy cooking.

F   A healthy portion of meat, poultry, or fish weighs six to eight ounces.

Short Answer

1. **What are the benefits of using standard recipes?**

   Standard recipes create consistency, make recipe costing easier and more accurate, reduce waste, and help to ensure that nutritional claims are adhered to.

2. **What types of recipes are not good candidates for modification?**

   Recipes that rely on fat for the majority of their flavor and texture are not good candidates.

3. **When modifying a recipe, what three variables may be adjusted?**

   Technique, ingredients, and portion size

3. **What pre-existing elements in a restaurant can be used as resources when taking a market survey?**

   Dining room staff and sales reports

4. **What customer traits should be considered in menu development?**

   Age, gender, and lifestyle should be taken into consideration.

5. **What are some techniques that can be used to make a healthy portion of meat, poultry, or fish appear larger?**

   Stuffing, cutting on the bias, slicing and fanning, and pounding or butterflying

Chapter Twelve:
Analyzing the Nutrient Content of Recipes

Objectives

After reading and studying this chapter, the student should be able to:
1.   Understand different methods of recipe analysis.
2.   Understand the variables relevant to recipe analysis.

Lecture Outline

Analyzing nutrient content
          Natural variables
          Processing and cooking
Methods of analysis
          Using recipes that have been previously analyzed
          Using food tables and labels
          Using a consultant
          Using computer software
Variables of analysis
          Exchanging information of like ingredients
          Preparation methods
          Making an educated guess
                    Marinades
                    Consommé rafts

Activities/Assignments

1. Using a nutrient value handbook, analyze a recipe by hand.

2. Select a recipe that requires ingredient value substitution or estimation and analyze it by hand or computer. Compare your results with others.

Sample Study and Test questions

Discussion Topics and Essay Questions

1. List and explain the variables that may affect nutritional analysis.

2. Explain the different ways to obtain nutritional analysis.

True/False

T   Nutritional analysis is required by the FDA if a restaurant makes nutritional or health claims about certain foods.

F   Nutritional analysis requires special training and costly computer software.

T   Nutrient values should be regarded only as an estimate.

F   If your ingredient handbook or database does not have a listing for an ingredient you are using, it is crucial that you obtain the correct values before proceeding.

T   If certain ingredients in a recipe, such as a marinade or mirepoix, are not entirely part of the finished product, it is acceptable to estimate how much will remain in the product for the purposes of nutritional analysis.

Short Answer

1. **Why is the nutritional analysis of foods only an estimate?**

   Natural variations occur in foods due to growing, storage, processing and cooking conditions.

2. **What are usually the most relevant values in recipe analysis?**

   Calories, fats, cholesterol, sodium, sugar and fiber are usually the most important values.

3. **What is the simplest way to obtain recipe analysis?**

   Use recipes that have already been analyzed.

4. **List the different ways nutritional analyses may be obtained.**

   Use recipes that have already been analyzed, analyze your own using reference tables and food labels or specially designed computer software, or hire a consultant to do the analyses for you.

5. **What are some of the ways you can ensure that dishes meet their nutritional standards?**

   Proper training of your kitchen staff and using standard recipes

Chapter Thirteen:
Nutrition Labeling in Menus and Advertisements

Objectives

After reading and studying this chapter, the student will be able to:
1. Understand the FDA guidelines for nutritional and health claims.
2. Understand the distinctions between different types of nutritional claims.

Lecture Outline

The history of nutritional legislation
        Packaged foods
        Restaurant menus
Nutrient content claims
        Reference amounts
        Absolute claim
        Relative claim
        Implied claim
Non-nutritional claims
Health claims
        FDA guidelines
        Nutrient/disease relationships
                Calcium and osteoporosis
                Fat and cancer
                Sodium and hypertension
                Saturated fat and cholesterol and risk of heart disease
                Fiber, fruits and vegetables and cancer
                Fruits, vegetables and grains with fiber and heart disease
                Folate and neural tube defects
                Dietary sugar and dental caries
                Soluble fiber from whole oats and coronary heart disease
Dietary guidelines

Activities/Assignments

1. Visit a local supermarket and survey products to see how nutrient labeling appears. Try to identify absolute, relative, and health claims. Try to find a dietary guideline statement on a product.

Keywords

Absolute claim-

Dietary guidelines-

Health claim-

Implied claim-

NLEA-

Nutrient content claim-

Reference amounts-

Relative claim-

Sample Study and Test Questions

Discussion Topics and Essay Questions

1. Define "nutrient content claim" and explain the three types outlined by the FDA.

2. What are health claims and how are they different from nutrient content claims?

3. Explain what it means for a food to be consistent with dietary guidelines.

True/False

T   According to a 1995 NRA report, 2/5 of all customers between the ages of 18 and 34 look for low-fat menu options.

F   The government does not regulate "low-fat" claims on a menu.

F   The FDA characterizes "low-sodium" as a relative claim.

T   Health claims are regulated by the FDA.

T   A health claim that involves dietary fat and cancer must be low fat.

F   A claim concerning dietary guidelines is a health claim.

Short Answer

1.   **What is the NLEA and why is its significant?**

      The NLEA is the Nutrition Labeling and Education Act. It requires virtually all

      packaged foods to have standardized nutritional labeling.

2.   **Explain what an absolute claim is according to the FDA.**

      An absolute claim gives an exact amount or range for a particular nutrient in a

      food. Examples are "low sodium" and "fat free."

3.   **What is a reference amount?**

      Reference amounts are standardized serving sizes set by the FDA that are used to

      calculate the nutrient content of foods.

4.   **What is a health claim?**

      Health claims refer to a nutrient substance in relation to a health-related issue.

5.   **How does the NLEA apply to foodservice operations?**

      Foodservice operators are not required to provide nutritional information. If they

      choose to do so, FDA labeling regulations apply to menus and advertising.

      Operators must have documentation to back any claims they make.

Chapter Fourteen:
Staff Training and Customer Communication

Objectives
After reading and studying this chapter, the student will be able to:
1. Understand the importance of training both dining room and kitchen staff.
2. Discuss the important points to consider when developing menu language for healthy cuisine.

Lecture Outline
Service staff
> How to speak to customers about healthy cuisine
> How to handle special requests
>> Preferences
>> Allergies
>> Dietary restrictions
> Maintaining lines of communication with kitchen staff

Kitchen staff
> Training
>> Cooking techniques
>> Standardized recipes
>> Preparation techniques
>> Handling questions from the service staff

Menu language

Communicating nutrition
> Type of establishment and clientele
>> Bistros and Executive Dining
>> Family Style Restaurants
>> Home Meal Replacement
>> Spas and Health Resorts
>> Institutional (Schools, Hospitals, etc.)

Activities/Assignments

1. Write a sample menu for a fine dining restaurant that uses descriptive language to emphasize health attributes of menu items.

2. When you visit various foodservice operations, make note of how they communicate nutrition, if at all, to you, the customer. Consider how effective these attempts are.

Sample Study and Test Questions

Discussion Topics and Essay Questions

1. Discuss why it is important to train dining room staff in handling special requests.

2. Discuss the importance of training kitchen staff in cooking and preparation techniques.

3. Explain why it is important to consider the type of restaurant when developing menu copy for healthy cuisine.

True/False

F When describing a low-fat dish to a customer, it is good practice for a server to leave out extra descriptions and just tell the customer that the dish is "low-fat."

F If a line cook puts a splash of extra oil in the pan, it will not have a significant effect on the overall nutritive value of the dish.

T Communication between the kitchen and dining room staff is vital.

T In healthy cooking, precise technique is of the utmost importance.

F Pre-service meetings should be held once a week.

Short Answer

1.   **How should servers be trained to handle special requests?**

They should be made aware of menu changes that are simple and complicated and they should know it is important to check with the appropriate people before making promises to customers.

2.   **What is the most effective way to communicate nutrition on a menu?**

There is no "best way." It varies according to the type of establishment and clientele.

3.   **Why is it important for the kitchen staff to be aware of the ingredients in prepared foods used in the kitchen?**

Prepared foods may contain an ingredient that a particular customer cannot or does not want to have in their food.

4.   **What is the fringe benefit of proper training?**

It raises employee self-esteem, resulting in improved productivity and reduced employee turnover.

5.   **List 2 methods that might be used by a fine-dining restaurant to communicate nutrition information to its customers.**

Server training, descriptive menu language, icons, referrals, healthy cooking demonstrations

Cooking Glossary

Á la minute: French for "to the minute." A restaurant production approach in which dishes are not prepared until an order arrives in the kitchen.

Allumette: Vegetables, potatoes or other items cut into pieces the size and shape of matchsticks, 1/8 inch x 1/8 inch x 1 to 2 inches is the standard.

Acidulated water: Water to which a small amount of lemon juice or other acid has been added. It is used to prevent discoloration of cut fruits and vegetables and as a cooking liquid.

Baguette: A loaf of bread shaped into a long cylinder.

Batch cooking: A cooking technique in which small batches of food are prepared several times throughout a service period so a fresh supply of cooked items is always available.

Batonnet: A stick-shaped vegetable cut in which pieces measure about 1/4 inch square and 2 to 2 1/2 inches long.

Blanch: To cook a food very briefly in order to remove strong odors, set the color, improve the texture, set the shape of the item, shorten the final preparation time, or make skins easier to remove.

Bloom: To rehydrate gelatin in a liquid before use.

Bouquet garni: A bunch of herbs, aromatics, and spices tied together inside celery stalks or leek leaves. The standard ingredients are parsley stems, a sprig of thyme, celery or leeks, and bay leaves.

Brunoise/small dice: A neat cut in which pieces are quite regular, about 1/8 inch on each side.

Carryover cooking: The cooking action of residual heat that remains in foods after they have been removed from the heat source.

Chiffonade: Leafy vegetables or herbs cut into fine shreds; often used as a garnish.

Clarification: The process of removing solid impurities from a liquid (such as butter or stock). Also, a mixture of ground meat, egg whites, mirepoix, tomato purée, herbs, and spices used to clarify broth for consommé.

Concassé / concasser (Fr.): To pound or chop coarsely. See also tomato concassé.

Confit: A preserve made by cooking the main ingredient (meat or vegetable) in a flavorful substance (typically, pork, goose and duck fat, but also ingredients such as honey, vinegar, or an extremely rich stock) until tender enough to spread easily.

Cordon: A ribbon of sauce ladled so that it surrounds the main item.

Coulis: A sauce (savory or sweet) made by puréeing the main ingredient to achieve a texture that ranges from very smooth to slightly coarse.

Court bouillon: "Short broth" in French. A vegetable-based broth that includes ingredients such as onions, thinly sliced carrots, celery, leeks, fresh herbs, spices, wine or vinegar; used to poach or steam foods.

Debeard: To remove the shaggy inedible fibers from a mussel. These fibers are used to anchor the mussel to its mooring.

Deglaze: To release the reduced drippings in a roasting or sauté pan by adding a liquid and stirring over heat.

Disjointed: Cut into pieces by cutting through the joints. Rabbits, chickens, crabs, and lobsters are often referred to as being "disjointed."

Dry-sauté: To sauté in a pan, usually nonstick, which has been coated with a thin film of oil.

Duxelles: A preparation made by sautéing a mixture of minced shallots, finely chopped mushrooms, white wine, and herbs until all liquids have been reduced. Duxelles is used as stuffing or as an ingredient in other preparations such as sauces or forcemeats.

Émince: A meat: cut in which lean meat is sliced into thin, regular strips.

Farro: An ancient unhybridized form of wheat known botanically as Triticum dicoccum. It has a hearty, nutty flavor and is traditionally eaten in the Tuscan region of Italy, often combined with cannellini beans.

Fermière: A disk-shaped vegetable cut into pieces that are sliced so that they retain their natural shape.

Fine brunoise/fine dice: A neat cut in which pieces are quite regular, about 1/16 inch on each side.

Fold: To gently mix together two items, usually a light airy mixture with a denser mixture.

Fond de veau (lié): A base sauce made by simmering browned veal bones, mirepoix, and a bouquet garni or sachet d'épices in brown veal stock. When thickened with a starch such as arrowroot, it is known as fond de veau lié.

Forcemeat: Meat which has been so finely ground that it achieves a soft, paste like consistency. The grinding action forces together lean meat with binders such as fat, cream, eggs, and/or starch-based ingredients such as rice.

Fortified wine: A wine to which a certain amount of alcohol and sugar has been added to increase the overall alcohol content. Marsala, Madeira, ports, and sherries are all examples.

Fumet: A stock made by allowing the major flavoring ingredient to cook with aromatics before the liquid is added to extract the greatest flavor in the shortest cooking time. Typically used for fish, shellfish, and vegetables.

Glace de viande (meat glaze): A meat-based stock which has been reduced to the point at which the texture becomes viscous and syrupy.

Gratin: Browned in an oven or under a broiler.

Infuse: To steep an aromatic or other item in liquid to extract its flavor.

Julienne: Vegetables, potatoes, or other items cut into thin strips; 1/8 inch square x 1 to 2 inches is standard. Fine julienne is 1/16-inch square.

Jus lié (Fr.): Meat juice thickened lightly with arrowroot or cornstarch.

Kasha: Toasted buckwheat groats.

Large dice: A neat cut in which pieces are quite regular, about 3/4 inch on each side.

Mark on a grill: To turn a food (without flipping it over), 90 degrees after it has been on the grill for several seconds to create the cross-hatch mark that is associated with grilled foods.

Medallion: A cut of meat, usually from the loin or tenderloin, shaped so that it has a neat, round shape and a uniform thickness.

Medium dice: A neat cut in which pieces are quite regular, about 1/3 inch on each side.

Mince: To chop into fine, fairly regular pieces.

Mirepoix: A combination of vegetables used to give flavor to various stocks, sauces, and gravies, as well as poached, simmered, braised, and stewed dishes. The standard ratio is two parts onion, one part carrot, one part celery.

Mise en place: French for "put in place." The preparation and assembly of ingredients, pans, utensils, and plates or serving pieces needed for a particular dish or service period.

Mousseline: A forcemeat with very fine texture.

Nage: A court bouillon or lightly flavored broth.

Oignon Brûlé (Fr.): "Burnt onion." A peeled, halved onion seared on a flat-top or a skillet and used to enhance the color and flavor of a stock or consommé.

Oignon Piqué (Fr.): "Pricked onion.":A whole, peeled onion to which a bay leaf is attached, using a whole clove as a tack. It is classically used to flavor béchamel sauce and some soups.

Pan-steam: To steam an item by placing it in a pan with a small amount of water or other liquid and heating it on a stove top.

Parcook: To partially cook an item before storing or finishing by another method; may be the same as blanching.

Parisienne: A cut prepared using a small melon baller, also known as a "parisienne" scoop.

Pluches: Herb leaves which are whole, left intact by a small bit of stem; often used as garnish.

Poach: A method in which items are cooked in a gently simmering liquid.

Poêlé: A method in which items are cooked in their own juices (usually with the addition of a matignon, other: aromatics, and melted butter) in a covered pot, usually in the oven.

Presentation side: The side of a piece of meat, poultry, or fish that will be served facing up.

Proof: To allow yeast dough to rise.

Purée: To chop an item extremely finely.

Quenelles: Small football-shaped dumplings traditionally shaped by molding a mixture with two spoons.

Raft: The sold mass that forms in a consommé when a clarification mixture has cooked long enough.

Ragoût: A stew.

Reduce: To cook a liquid long enough to reduce its original volume, concentrating the flavor, color, and body of the original item.

Remouillage: A second stock made from bones which have already been used to prepare a stock. This "second wetting" is frequently used either to prepare glace de viande or as the liquid to prepare subsequent batches of stock.

Ribbon cut: A neat, regular cut in which foods are cut into extremely thin strips.

Rondeau: A shallow, wide, straight-sided pot with two loop handles.

Rough chop: To cut foods into fairly regular pieces. The dimensions can vary according to the overall cooking time required; the longer the cooking time, the larger the piece.

Roulade: A rolled item. Meats which are filled, rolled, and tied into cylinders are referred to as roulades, as are sponge cakes which are filled and rolled.

Roux: A traditional thickener made by cooking together flour and butter. (Oil or other fats may be used to replace butter).

Sachet d'épices: A cheesecloth parcel of herbs and spices (usually dried) used to infuse a simmered or poached dish with a special flavor. A standard sachet usually includes parsley stems, dried thyme leaves, bay leaves, and cracked peppercorns. Other ingredients may be added as desired.

Semolina: The coarsely milled hard wheat endosperm used for gnocchi, couscous, and some pasta and breads.

Score: To cut the surface of an item at regular intervals to allow it to cook evenly.

Slurry: Starch dispersed in cold liquid to prevent it from forming lumps when added to hot liquid as a thickener.

Smoke-roasting: A method for roasting foods in which items are placed on a rack in a pan containing wood chips that smolder, emitting smoke, when the pan is placed on the range top or in the oven.

Smoking point: The temperature at which fats start to break down when heated.

Smother: To cook something over gentle heat in enough liquid or fat to barely cover it, until it begins to release its own essence.

Steep: To allow an ingredient to sit in warm or hot liquids to extract flavor or impurities, or to soften the item.

Stock: A basic element in a kitchen's mise en place made by simmering flavorful ingredients in water to extract flavor and color.

Supreme: The breast of a bird (domestic or game) in which bones have been removed, with the exception of one portion of the wing bone. That section is scraped free of all meat and sinew, and is referred to as "frenched."

Sweat: To cook a food (especially aromatic vegetables) over low heat in a small amount of a flavorful liquid or stock with a cover on the pot until it releases its own juices.

Terrine: A forcemeat-based loaf, traditionally baked in an earthenware dish.

Timbale: A small mold, usually taller than wide, used to prepare custards or other dishes, also used to refer to dishes prepared in these molds.

Tomato concassé: Peeled, seeded tomatoes which have been chopped, julienned, or cut into dice.

Tourné: A barrel-shaped vegetable cut, usually with seven sides

Tuiles/tiles: Thin wafer-like cookies (or foods cut to resemble these cookies). Tuiles and tiles are frequently "shaped" while still pliable by pressing them into molds or draping them over rolling pins or dowels.

Umami: Japanese word that describes a savory, meaty taste; often associated with monosodium glutamate (MSG).

Velouté: A sauce made by thickening stock. Traditionally made by simmering stocks with roux; in healthy cooking roux is replaced by arrowroot.

Vinaigrette: A cold sauce made by forming an emulsion of oil and vinegar in a specific ratio. Traditional vinaigrette calls for 3 parts oil and 1 part vinegar; in healthy cooking, the majority of the oil is replaced with a thickened stock.

White mirepoix: A mirepoix in which the carrots are either omitted or replaced by parsnips. Frequently leeks are used to replace some of the onions as well.

Nutrition Glossary

Absolute claim: A type of nutrient content claim that characterizes the exact amount or range of a nutrient in a particular food.

Additives: Substances added to foods to help preserve them, as well as to improve nutritive value, palatability, and eye appeal. Additives fall into many categories including emulsifiers, flavorings, thickeners, curing agents, stabilizers, coloring agents, nutrients, and inhibitors (which act against molds, yeasts and bacteria). Permissible amounts of most additives are subject to government regulation.

Amino acid: A compound composed of hydrogen, carbon, oxygen, and nitrogen, the amino acid is the building block of all proteins. There are 20 to 22 amino acids used to produce all of the protein found in the human body: 8 must be supplied in the diet (9 for infants and small children). See also essential amino acids.

Antioxidants: Substances that retard the breakdown of tissues in the presence of oxygen. May be added to food during processing, or may be naturally-occurring. As an example, many fats, especially vegetable oils, contain Vitamin E, which acts to protect the oils from becoming rancid for a limited period of time.

Appetite: A learned or habitual response to a variety of stimuli that encourages a person to eat. The cues which encourage appetite may be internal (onset of real hunger, drop in blood sugar) or external (sights and smells of appealing foods).

Arteriosclerosis: A condition in which fibrous tissue and fatty deposits build up on the artery walls, causing thickening and loss of elasticity. This is one of the risk factors associated with the development of cardiovascular diseases.

Atherosclerosis: A type of arteriosclerosis in which fatty deposits have caused the walls of the arteries to dramatically thicken, constricting the passageway so that the blood supply to the heart and brain is reduced to the point that there is danger of coronary heart disease or stroke.

Basal metabolism: The amount of energy, expressed in calories, required by the body at rest to carry on all the necessary involuntary functions to sustain life (breathing, digestion, heart beat, etc.)

Blood pressure: A measurement of the pressure exerted by blood flowing through the arteries. Expressed in both systolic and diastolic pressure, which represent the pressure as the heart pumps, and as it relaxes, respectively.

Calorie (Kilocalorie, Kcal, or Calorie): The amount of heat necessary to raise the temperature of a kilogram (liter) of water 1 degree Centigrade. It is a measure of the energy supplied in foods.

Carbohydrate: The term is derived from "carbo" (carbon) and "hydrate" (water) reflecting the components of all carbohydrates: carbon, oxygen, and hydrogen. It is the source of energy preferred by the body. Carbohydrates include simple carbohydrates (also known as simple sugars) and complex carbohydrates (referred to as starch or fiber). Simple carbohydrates are generally formed from one or two sugars (referred to as mono- or di-saccharide), which may be naturally-occurring (those found in fruits or milk), or refined (added sugars, including honey, table sugar, molasses, and corn syrup).

Carotenoids: Antioxidant pigments found in yellow, orange, red, and leafy green vegetables.

Cholesterol: A fatty acid, belonging to a group known as the sterols, a category of lipid (the general term for fats of all types). Essential to hormone production, creation of cell membranes, acts as protection for nerve fibers, responsible for production of Vitamin D on the skin's surface in the presence of sunlight. See also dietary cholesterol and serum (blood) cholesterol.

Complementary proteins: A combination of foods, each of which supplies varying amounts of different amino acids so that the amino acids lacking or in insufficient supply in one food are complemented by those found in the second food.

Complete proteins: A food source that provides all of the essential amino acids in the correct ratio so that they can be used in the body for protein synthesis.

Complex carbohydrates: Long chains composed of many sugars, referred to as polysaccharides. One of the forms of complex carbohydrates is starch, which is the plant's storage system that holds energy to support future growth. The other is fiber, the structural component of plants. These carbohydrates may be found in foods as they naturally occur (whole grains or whole-grain meals and flours) or they may be refined during the processes of polishing and bleaching.

Conditionally essential amino acid: An amino acid that can be produced by the body from the essential amino acids under normal circumstances; when essential amino acids are not consumed in sufficient amounts, a dietary source is necessary for conditionally essential amino acids.

Daily Values (DVs): Standard values developed by the Food and Drug Administration (FDA) for use on food labels. In creating the Daily Values, the FDA first established two sets of reference values. The first set, the Reference Daily Intakes (RDI), are for protein, vitamins, and minerals and reflect average allowances based on the RDA (see Recommended Dietary Allowances). The second set, the Daily Reference Values (DRV), are for nutrients and food components, such as fat and fiber, that do not have an established RDA but do have important relationships with health. Together, the RDI and DRV make up the Daily Values used on food labels.

Denaturation: A change in the structure of a protein brought about by applying heat, an acid, a base, or by agitation.

Dietary cholesterol: The cholesterol found in the foods included as part of the diet. Only found in land and sea animals. Egg yolks, most organ meats, and some shellfish are especially high in dietary cholesterol. Some individuals experience a sensitivity to dietary cholesterol.

Empty calories: Calories provided by a food or beverage with either a very limited number of nutrients or none at all in comparison to their caloric content.

Energy nutrients: The substances found in foods that can be broken down in the body, and used for energy, as well as for the growth, repair, and replacement of tissues. These nutrients include carbohydrates, protein, and fat.

Enrichment: Addition of lost nutrients to a processed food. These nutrients are naturally present in whole foods, but are lost during processing or refining. Some or all of the lost nutrients may be replaced.

Epinephrine: The hormone that converts glycogen into glucose. Also known as adrenaline.

Essential amino acid: One of the amino acids that the body requires but cannot produce itself. There are 8 amino acids required by adults. Small children and infants required an additional amino acid. All of the essential amino acids must be supplied, in the correct ratios, in order for the body to produce the proteins necessary for health.

Essential nutrients: Compounds needed by the body which must be supplied through the diet. Includes water, vitamins, minerals, carbohydrates, proteins, and fats. Although fiber does not supply the body with nutrients, since it cannot be digested, it is another essential component of a healthy diet.

Fat: One of the essential nutrients. Fat supplies the body with essential fatty acids as well as being the most concentrated source of energy. Fats are solid (or plastic) at room temperature; oils are liquid.

Fatty acid: The basic chemical unit of fats; composed of carbon, hydrogen, and oxygen.

Fermentation: The effect produced by compounds that act on various substances to transform them or metabolize them in the absence of oxygen. For example, sugar is fermented by enzymes in yeast to form carbon dioxide and alcohol during bread baking.

Fiber: The portion of plant foods composed of complex carbohydrates. Soluble fiber is the pectin and gums found in whole grains, fruits and vegetables; insoluble fiber is lignin and hemicellulose found in whole grains, fruits, and vegetables. Fiber cannot be digested by humans.

Fortification: The addition of nutrients, typically vitamins and minerals, that were not originally present in the food. Examples include the addition of iodine to salt, calcium to flour, and Vitamins A or D to skim milk.

Gluten: The protein found in flours, especially wheat flour that is capable of forming the elastic strands that enable yeast-leavened to rise by stretching enough to trap the gases released during fermentation.

Glycogen: The form in which the body stores carbohydrate in the liver and in muscle tissue to be available for use when glucose stores are depleted.

Gram: A gram (abbreviated as GM) is the weight of one cubic centimeter (or milliliter) of water under specifically defined conditions of temperature and pressure.

Health claim: A statement that characterizes the relationship between the nutrient content of a foods and a disease or health-related condition.

Healthy Body Weight (abbreviated as HBW): A weight determined by using any of a number of calculations that is considered "best" for an individual. Usually this weight is based on a number of factors measured by health care providers or fitness experts, including percentage of body fat in relation to lean muscle mass, activity level, age, gender, and overall health and fitness conditions. The weight calculated in this way may be above or below the "ideal" body weight values given in standard insurance charts or "reasonable" body weight calculated by using a standard formula based on height, frame size, and activity level.

High-Density Lipoprotein (HDL): Clusters of lipids associated with protein particles capable of transporting fats through the bloodstream. HDL has a higher protein content than other lipoprotein in relation to its fat content. HDL is sometimes referred to as the "good cholesterol." Its function appears to be the return of cholesterol from storage areas to the liver so that it can be dismantled and eliminated from the body. See also Low-Density Lipoprotein (LDL).

Homogenization: A mechanical process that forces mixtures of fats and other liquids through a fine mesh to make fat globules smaller and of approximately the same size so that they will disperse evenly and will not separate out of the mixture and rise to the top.

Hydrogenation: The process of forcing hydrogen to bond at open sites in a mono- or polyunsaturated oil to produce a product that is more solid at room temperature.

Shortenings and margarines are examples of hydrogenated fats. Once hydrogenated, a fat becomes more saturated than it was originally, though it may still be considered predominantly unsaturated. Hydrogenation results in the formation of trans fats.

Hypertension: The term used to indicate chronic elevated blood pressure. This condition is often associated with atherosclerosis, obesity, inactivity, and diets high in sodium and fats.

Implied claim: A type of nutrient content claim that highlights the presence or absence of a particular ingredient that is known to be associated with the level of a particular nutrient.

Incomplete protein: A protein found in plant foods that is either entirely lacking one or more of the essential amino acids, or had a supply that is small enough that it cannot be used by the body to promote the growth, repair, or replacement of body tissue. The deficiency can be compensated for by eating a variety of foods throughout the day that will supply adequate amounts of all the essential amino acids.

Ketones: Toxic by-products that are formed when fats are broken down incompletely in the body.

Ketosis: The potentially harmful state that results when ketones accumulate in the body.

Kilocalorie: See Calorie.

Lipids: The name given to family of substances that includes triglycerides (known as fats and oils), phospholipids (lecithin is an example), and sterols (the most familiar is cholesterol). These compounds are essential to the body, and are found throughout the food supply as well as being produced by the body. Those produced in the body are usually known as "blood" or "serum" cholesterol or triglycerides.

Low-Density Lipoprotein (LDL): Clusters of lipids associated with protein particles capable of transporting fats through the bloodstream. LDL has a lower protein content than high-density lipoprotein in relation to its fat content. LDL is usually associated with an increased risk of heart disease. Its function is the transport of cholesterol from the liver to other body cells.

Macro mineral (major mineral): An essential mineral nutrient that is found in the human body in amounts greater than five grams.

Metabolism: The total of all chemical reactions that occur in living cells. These reactions convert food into an energy source that the body can use.

Micro mineral (trace mineral): An essential mineral nutrient found in the body in amounts less than five grams.

Mineral: An organic compound that is an essential component of the diet. Provides no energy, and is therefore referred to as a non-caloric nutrient.

Monosodium glutamate: The sodium salt of glutamic acid; used as a seasoning and flavor enhancer.

Monounsaturated fat: A fat or oil that is composed of fatty acids that have one point that is not bonded with hydrogen. Oils which have a high proportion of monounsaturated fats tend to be flavorful; examples include oils found in or produced from avocados, olives, and most nuts.

Mutual supplementation: The process of consuming various incomplete complementary protein sources to supply all essential amino acids.

Nutrient content claim: A statement regarding the nutrition profile of foods.

Nutrient dense: Describes a food source that has a good supply of nutrients in relation to the number of calories it contains.

Nutrients: Compounds required by the body in order to maintain life. The six classes of nutrients (known as the essential nutrients) include carbohydrates, fat, protein, vitamins, minerals, and water.

Olestra: A fat substitute based on an altered form of fat and carbohydrate that is not absorbed by the body.

Oligosaccharides: Indigestible complex sugars found in high fiber foods.

Omega-3 fatty acids: Polyunsaturated fatty acids that may reduce the risk of heart disease and tumor growth, stimulate the immune system, and lower blood pressure; they occur in fatty fish, dark green leafy vegetables, and certain nuts and oils.

Osteoporosis: A health condition of deteriorated bone mass, or density.

Pasteurize: To preserve and/or sanitize foods by heating them at a sufficient temperature for a specified length of time in order to destroy certain microorganisms and to arrest fermentation. the exact temperature and length of time required varies from food to food. Milk and certain fruit juices are routinely pasteurized.

Phytochemicals: Naturally-occurring compounds in plant foods that have antioxidant and disease-fighting properties.

Polyunsaturated fat: A chain of fatty acids in which two or more points are not filled with a hydrogen atom. Oils composed predominantly of polyunsaturated fats are often of plant origin, liquid at room temperature, with a neutral flavor. They are found in, or refined from, corn, safflower, and cottonseed.

Protein: A compound formed by carbon, hydrogen, oxygen, and nitrogen when arranged into strands of amino acids. One of the six categories of essential nutrients Found in a variety of food sources, including meats, milk and dairy products, eggs, grains, vegetables, and legumes.

Protein-sparing: The condition whereby carbohydrates and fat supply sufficient stores of energy so that protein is able to perform other vital functions: growth, maintenance, and repair of tissue.

Recommended Dietary Allowances (RDA): Suggested level of a variety of nutrients prepared by the Food and Nutrition Board (FNB) of the National Academy of Sciences/National Research Council (NAS/NRC). Separate recommendations are made for different sets of healthy people, grouped by age and gender. All recommendations include a substantial margin of safety and are not to be considered minimum requirements for healthy individuals.

Refined sugars: Sugars made by concentrating and purifying simple carbohydrates found in other foods (honey, table sugar, molasses, corn syrup, etc.).

Relative claim: A type of nutrient content claim that characterizes the nutrient content of one food compared to another.

Satiety: the feeling of fullness or satisfaction after eating. Fat is capable of providing a more lasting sense of fullness, since it is digested last, and more slowly, than other nutrients.

Saturated fat: A chain of fatty acids in which all available sites for hydrogen bonds are full. Fats that are composed predominantly of saturated fats tend to be solid at room temperature and of animal origin. The "tropical oils" including coconut, palm, and palm kernel oils are exceptions to both of the preceding general statements. Saturated fats are associated with an increase in serum cholesterol levels.

Serum cholesterol: Cholesterol found in the bloodstream. May also be referred to as "blood cholesterol." Carried by lipoproteins, this cholesterol is generally produced in the body from the triglycerides provided by a diet high in saturated fats.

Simple carbohydrates: Also known as sugars, which may be single (monosaccharides) or double (disaccharides). These sugars are either "naturally-occurring" (e.g., fructose found in fruit) or "refined sugars" (e.g., sucrose found in table sugar).

Simple sugars: See Carbohydrate.

Trans fat: A type of fatty acid that is formed when unsaturated fats are hydrogenated (trans fats also occur naturally in foods). Trans fats may have an effect on serum cholesterol levels similar to saturated fats.

Vegetarian: An individual who has adopted a specific diet (or lifestyle) that reduces or eliminated all sources of animal products. Vegans eat no foods derived in any way from animals (some even exclude honey); lacto-ovo vegetarians include eggs and dairy products in their diet. Other people refer to themselves as "vegetarians" but will occasionally eat fish or poultry, preferring to exclude only red meats.

Vitamin: An organic compound considered an essential nutrient. Vitamins provide no energy, and are referred to as non-caloric nutrients. They may be water-soluble or fat-soluble.

Water: One of the six essential nutrients. Water provides no calories and is vital to the proper function of the body.

Transparency Masters

THE SEVEN PRINCIPLES OF HEALTHY COOKING

1. **Select ingredients with care.**
   - Design menus to include a large variety of ingredients.
   - Emphasize high-quality ingredients.
   - Use fresh, seasonal produce in menu planning when reasonable.
   - Explore nontraditional ingredients for providing the function and flavor of traditional high-fat, high-sodium ingredients.

2. **Store and prepare all foods with the aim of preserving their best possible flavor, texture, color, and overall nutritional value.**
   - Control temperatures carefully in receiving, storage, preparation, and service.
   - Select and execute fundamental cooking techniques properly to ensure quality finished products.

3. **Incorporate a variety of plant-based dishes on the menu in all categories.**
   - Shift the emphasis toward grains, legumes, vegetables, and fruits.
   - For inspiration, look to traditional ethnic cuisines that are predominantly plant-based.

4. **Manage the amount of fat used both as an ingredient and as part of a preparation or cooking technique.**
   - Opt for unsaturated vegetable oils whenever possible and reduce the use of animal fats.
   - Select lean animal products and trim visible fats.
   - Use fat-dense foods (cream, butter, cheeses) sparingly.
   - Explore nontraditional, low-fat ingredients and methods.

5. **Serve appropriate portions of foods.**
   - Size portions to reflect the recommendations of the food guide pyramids.
   - Monitor overall menu balance; individual menu items may vary from the established guidelines as long as the entire menu is nutritionally balanced.

6. **Use salt with care and purpose.**
   - Explore a variety of seasonings, preparation methods, and cooking techniques to reduce reliance on salt.
   - Emphasize clean, distinct, assertive flavors.
   - Use high-sodium ingredients sparingly to add flavor.
   - Incorporate contemporary sauces, such as juices, salsas, and reductions, to increase flavor.

7. **Offer a variety of beverages, both alcoholic and nonalcoholic, that complement the food menu.**
   - Make the beverage menu as varied and interesting as the food menu.

TAKE TIME FOR SUCCESS

The Ten Commandments of the Kitchen

1. TAKE TIME TO THINK.
You will find this is the shortest, surest way to success. It avoids many costly mistakes. Think; you will find your work more interesting and less tiring.

2. TAKE TIME TO PLAN.
Plan your work in an orderly way and you will find work goes more smoothly, not only for you but also for every fellow worker.

3. TAKE TIME TO LISTEN.
You will not learn while you are talking. Listen and acquire knowledge. Listen and become popular with your fellow workers and guests. By listening, you let people know you are interested in them, their ideas, and their problems.

4. TAKE TIME TO PRAISE.
Go out of your way to compliment anyone for an outstanding job. This is the spirit that makes people want to succeed by making them want to try harder.

5. TAKE TIME TO SAY THANK YOU.
Go out of your way to say thank you to fellow workers and guests when they do something for you. Everyone appreciates it, and it will make you feel good too.

6. TAKE TIME TO SMILE.
Smile when you give instructions or when talking to a guest. It is the best way to win friends and cooperation.

7. TAKE TIME TO EXPLAIN.
When talking to others about their work, be specific and clear. Say just what you mean, and give the reason why. We all do our best when we understand what is expected of us.

8. TAKE TIME TO GIVE ORDERS CHEERFULLY.
Everyone who works has to take or give orders. We all respond better when they are given cheerfully.

9. TAKE TIME TO DO IT NOW.
Do not put things off. The longer you do, the more difficult the job becomes. Let people know they can depend on you to get things done.

10. TAKE TIME TO BE ENTHUSIASTIC.
Enthusiasm is contagious. Do everything with enthusiasm. You will find it an inspiration to your whole organization.

CHECKLIST FOR DESIRABLE WORK HABITS IN THE KITCHEN

Check yourself, improve yourself, then set an example for co-workers.

Do I wash my hands and see that my nails are clean before working?	YES	NO	SOMETIMES
Do I dry my hands only on paper towels, *not* my apron?	YES	NO	SOMETIMES
Do I keep my handkerchief put away while working? Or if it is necessary to use it, do I wash my hands again before working with food?	YES	NO	SOMETIMES
Do I wear a clean apron while working?	YES	NO	SOMETIMES
Am I getting all the supplies from the place of storage in as few trips as possible?	YES	NO	SOMETIMES
Am I shortening the work of cleaning by placing soiled utensils or scraps on a tray or paper towel or by working with my cutting board in a tray?	YES	NO	SOMETIMES
Do I use the smallest number of utensils necessary in cooking?	YES	NO	SOMETIMES
Do I use the most appropriate utensils for the foods I prepare?	YES	NO	SOMETIMES
Do I always use a clean utensil for tasting food, never use my fingers or the same utensil twice?	YES	NO	SOMETIMES
Do I use a piece of paper, cheesecloth, or a brush when greasing pans instead of my fingers?	YES	NO	SOMETIMES
Do I always use potholders to handle hot dishes and pans or at least a dry towel instead of a wet towel?	YES	NO	SOMETIMES
Do I save motions when washing dishes by keeping soiled dishes in one area and clean dishes in another?	YES	NO	SOMETIMES
Do I wash and dry knives and small utensils immediately?	YES	NO	SOMETIMES
Do I immediately wipe up grease or water that I have spilled or splattered?	YES	NO	SOMETIMES
Do I work quietly, without talking too much or too loudly?	YES	NO	SOMETIMES

COMPOSED SALAD COMPOSITION WORKSHEET

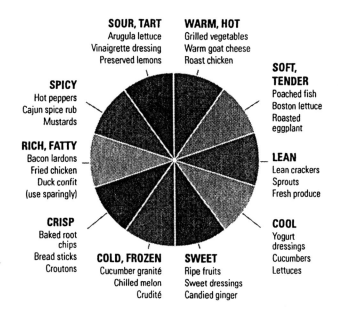

SOUR, TART
Arugula lettuce
Vinaigrette dressing
Preserved lemons

WARM, HOT
Grilled vegetables
Warm goat cheese
Roast chicken

SOFT, TENDER
Poached fish
Boston lettuce
Roasted eggplant

SPICY
Hot peppers
Cajun spice rub
Mustards

LEAN
Lean crackers
Sprouts
Fresh produce

RICH, FATTY
Bacon lardons
Fried chicken
Duck confit
(use sparingly)

COOL
Yogurt dressings
Cucumbers
Lettuces

CRISP
Baked root chips
Bread sticks
Croutons

COLD, FROZEN
Cucumber granité
Chilled melon
Crudité

SWEET
Ripe fruits
Sweet dressings
Candied ginger

Components	Flavors	Textures
Greens		
Main Items(s)		
Garnish(es)		
Dressing		

PLATED APPETIZER COMPOSITION WORKSHEET

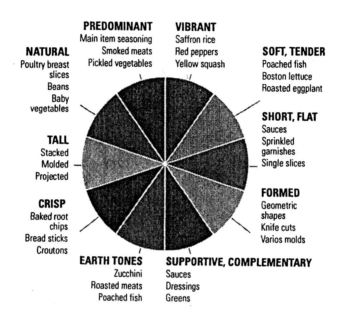

PREDOMINANT
Main item seasoning
Smoked meats
Pickled vegetables

VIBRANT
Saffron rice
Red peppers
Yellow squash

NATURAL
Poultry breast
slices
Beans
Baby
vegetables

SOFT, TENDER
Poached fish
Boston lettuce
Roasted eggplant

TALL
Stacked
Molded
Projected

SHORT, FLAT
Sauces
Sprinkled
garnishes
Single slices

CRISP
Baked root
chips
Bread sticks
Croutons

FORMED
Geometric
shapes
Knife cuts
Varios molds

EARTH TONES
Zucchini
Roasted meats
Poached fish

SUPPORTIVE, COMPLEMENTARY
Sauces
Dressings
Greens

Components	Flavor	Shape	Textures	Height	Color
Main Items(s)					
Accompaniment(s)					
Sauce					
Crisp					
Leaf (greens)					

KNIFE CUTS

It should be noted that these dimensions are recommended guidelines and are used to stress consistency and develop discipline for your knife skills. In common practice, professional chefs may not measure exactly to these guidelines. However, in most circumstances consistency will be expected.   **(Drawings are shown actual size.)**

JULIENNE
1/16" x 1/16" x 1" to 2"

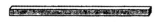

ALLUMETTE*
1/8" x 1/8" x 1" to 2 "

*This cut technically refers only to the cutting of potatoes 1/4" x 1/4" x 2"

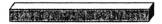

BATONNET
1/4" x 1/4" x 2" to 2 ½"

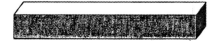

BRUNOISE
1/8" x 1/8" x 1/8"

SMALL DICE
1/4" x 1/4" x 1/4"

MEDIUM DICE
1/2" x 1/2" x 1/2"

LARGE DICE
3/4" x 3/4" x 3/4"

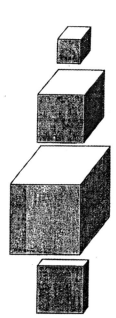

PAYSANNE
1/2" x 1/2" x 1/8"

TOURNÉ
2" x 7 even sides

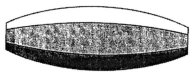

COOLING STOCKS

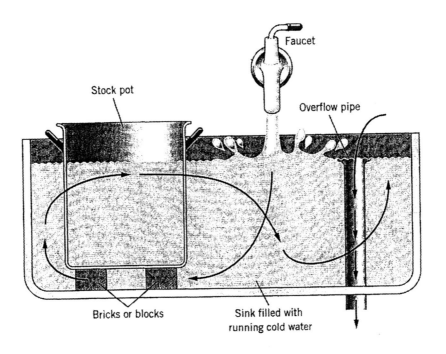

Stock pot

Faucet

Overflow pipe

Bricks or blocks

Sink filled with
running cold water

CONSOMMÉ

The Stages of Consommé during Clarification

1ˢᵗ Stage   **2ⁿᵈ Stage**   **3ʳᵈ Stage**

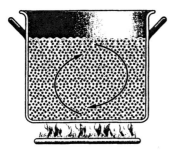   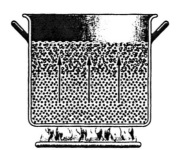   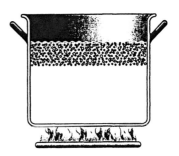

Consommé just after
being placed on the fire
(ingredients move freely)

Proteins begin to coagulate
and float to surface

Raft is formed on surface
and continues to shrink

ROASTING

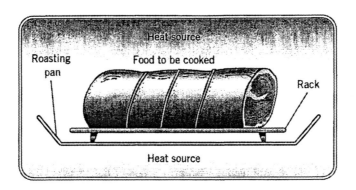

The Pros and Cons of Roasting

Pros	Cons
Food is cooked on a rack allowing the rendering fat to drip from food.	Tender, more expensive cuts of meat are used.
Foods receive flavor from caramelization.	Meat must have sufficient marbling or it will dry when roasted.
Better method for large cuts of meat.	

ROASTING TIPS:
- Flavor food with marinades.
- Use herbs and spices for seasonings.
- Serve with jus or jus liés.
- Trim excess fat before cooking.
- Roast meats on a rack to allow rendered fat to drain away from meat.

BROILERS AND GRILLS

BROILER

- Heat source radiates from above
- Limited conduction from the heat of the grids

Types of Broilers:

- Gas
- Electric

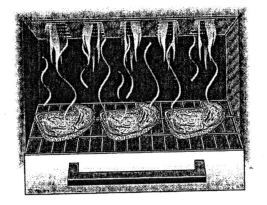

GRILL

- Heat source radiates from below
- Conduction and radiation of heat

Types of Grills:

- Gas
- Charcoal
- Hardwood

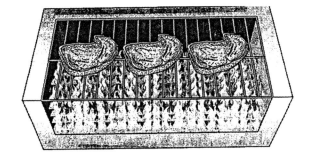

SAUTÉ

Sauté is a French verb meaning "to leap or jump." This translation, however, has little to do with the sautéing of most meat and seafood items. Because it does not translate easily into English, the word has become part of our culinary vocabulary just as other French words (maitre d'hôtel, garde manger) have. In culinary usage, "sauté" means to cook quickly in a small amount of fat. Traditionally, sautéing is done on top of the stove, but may be finished in a moderate oven. Sautéed items are cooked to order and are usually served with a pan sauce.

PANS USED FOR SAUTÉING

A shallow pan is used for sautéing because it allows moisture to escape. If moisture is trapped in the pan it causes the food to steam, toughening the meat and preventing browning.

Sauteuse (Sauté pan): Shallow pan with sloping sides.

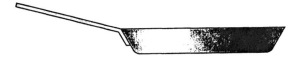

Sautoir: Shallow pan with straight sides.

In sautéing the following are required:

- A hot pan with a small amount of fat
- Thin tender food items with excess moisture blotted off
- Correct size pan for the amount of food to be cooked
- All mise en place required for preparing the item

SAUTÉ

Incorrect

The pan is overcrowded, trapping steam, which will prevent the meat from browning and cause the meat fibers to toughen.

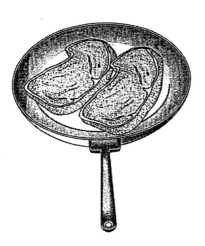

Correct

The pan is full but there is sufficient space between the pieces of meat, allowing steam to escape and prevent toughening.

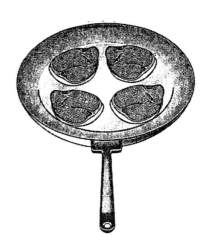

POACHING, SIMMERING, AND BOILING

Poaching, simmering, and boiling all cook foods in the same way, i.e. in liquid, and are therefore known as moist-heat methods. The liquid may be water, stock, or a sauce. It is the temperature of the liquid that marks the difference between the three methods.

Poaching	160°F to 180°F
Simmering	185°F to 200°F
Boiling	212°F +

Descriptions of the progression of the rising temperature of 2 quarts of water, with and without salt:

2 quarts water		2 quarts water + salt (1 to 4 ½ tablespoons.)
Minute bubbles adhere to sides and bottom of pan	140°F	Cloudiness occurs with 3 tablespoons or more of salt
Same as above with increase of bubble quantity	150°F	The use of salt between 140°F and 185°F eliminates the small and minute bubbles
Minute bubbles begin to break from bottom	160°F	
Bubbles begin to increase in size	170°F	
Increased size of bubbles with large quantities of bubbles coming to surface	180°F	
Increase of large bubble quantity with condensed packages of bubbles	190°F	Large bubbles coming to surface with increase in bubble quantity
Minimal agitation caused by bubbles	195°F	Large bubbles forming on bottom and breaking, like flashes
Very rapid dispersion of bubbles; agitation around sides	200°F	Release of steam; water appears to roll.
Surface agitation, mostly on sides with very rapid release of bubbles of large size and quantity	205°F	Movement on sides; large bubble with small bubbles on bottom surfacing with agitation
Very rapid release of large bubbles; beginning of a rolling agitation	210°F	Increase of large bubbles beginning to roll gently
Rapid rolling boil	212°F	Gentle rolling boil
	213°F 215°F	High rapid boil using 3 to 4 ½ tablespoons salt

SHALLOW VS. DEEP POACHING

Cross-section view of poaching techniques.

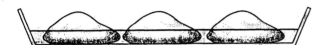

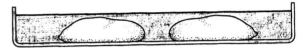

Shallow Poaching   Deep Poaching

Differences in Poaching Techniques

Shallow Poaching	Deep Poaching
Less liquid is used	More liquid is used
Appropriate for smaller cuts of meat, poultry, or fish	Appropriate for larger cuts of meat, poultry, or fish
A sauce is made from the poaching liquid	The poaching liquid is not used for the sauce; a separately derived sauce is used
Generally done in the oven	Generally done on top of the stove
The garnish may be included during the cooking	The garnish is cooked separately and added just before serving
The pan is covered with a paper cover	The pan is not covered

SHALLOW POACHING

160°F to 180°F

CORRECT SPACING FOR SHALLOW-POACHED FOODS

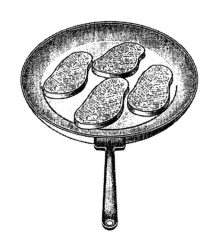

Descriptions of water at the following temperatures:

140°F	Minute bubbles adhere to sides and bottom of pan
150°F	Same as above with increase of bubble quantity
160°F	Minute bubbles begin to break from bottom
170°F	Bubbles begin to increase in size
180°F	Increased size of bubbles with large quantities of bubbles coming to surface

In shallow poaching the following are required:

- Shallow, wide pan

- Tender portion-size items

- Liquid maintained at a very slow simmer during cooking

- Sauce is made from the poaching liquid

- All mise en place required for preparing the item

SHALLOW POACHING

INCORRECT

The pan is too large causing you to add too much liquid to bring the liquid up the right level in the pan or causing the cuisson to evaporate too quickly and caramelize.

CORRECT

The pan is full but there is sufficient space between the fillets. This should cause you to put in an appropriate amount of poaching liquid.

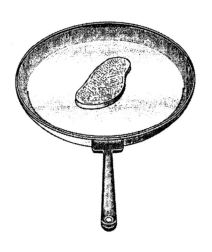 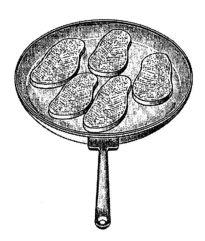

SIMMERING

A pot that is taller than it is wide is used to simmer various foods. The shape of the pot prevents excess evaporation.

Descriptions of water at the following temperatures:

190°F	Increase of large bubble quantity with condensed packages of bubbles
195°F	Minimal agitation caused by bubbles
200°F	Very rapid dispersion of bubbles; agitation around sides
205°F	Surface agitation, mostly on sides with very rapid release of bubbles of large size and quantity

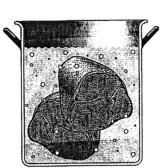

In simmering the following are required:

- Tall, narrow pot

- Tougher, more mature cuts of meat or poultry

- Liquid maintained at a gentle simmer during cooking

BOILING

The pot used for boiling should provide a large surface area.

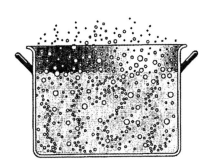

Descriptions of water at the following temperatures:

210°F	Very rapid release of large bubbles; beginning of a rolling agitation
212°F	Rapid rolling boil
212°F +	Adding salt to the water will increase the temperature at which water boils

In boiling the following are required:

- Large pot, plenty of water

- Food item – vegetables and pasta are the most commonly boiled foods

- Salt in water (optional)

- Water maintained at a rolling boil during cooking

- Cold water if shocking is required after boiling